Fortune Brown is a writer, blogger, researcher and a co-founder at www.wommenhealth.me. She is passionate about women health and personal care and wellness. She is happily married to a loving husband and blessed with two lovely boys.

TABLE OF CONTENT

LEGAL DISCLAIMER

This disclaimer governs the use of this book/eBook. By using this book, you accept this disclaimer in full. The information in this book reflects the author's opinion and is not intended to replace medical advice.

The author has made every effort to supply accurate information in the creation of this book. The author offers no warranty and accepts no responsibility for any loss or damages of any kind that may be incurred by the result of actions arising from the use of this book.

This ebook contains information about Getting Pregnant. The information is not a medical advice, and should not be treated as such.

You must not rely on the information in the ebook as an alternative to medical advice from an appropriately qualified professional. If you have any specific questions about any medical matter you should consult an appropriately qualified medical professional.

If you think you may be suffering from any medical condition you should seek immediate medical attention. You should never delay seeking medical advice, disregard medical advice, or discontinue medical treatment because of information in the ebook.

Without prejudice to the generality of the foregoing paragraph, we do not represent, warrant, undertake or guarantee:
    * that the information in the ebook is correct, accurate,

complete or non-misleading;

* that the use of the guidance in the ebook will lead to any particular outcome or result; or
*   in particular, that by using the guidance in the ebook you will get pregnant

If a section of this disclaimer is determined by any court or other competent authority to be unlawful and/or unenforceable, the other sections of this disclaimer continue in effect.

If any unlawful and/or unenforceable section would be lawful or enforceable if part of it were deleted, that part will be deemed to be deleted, and the rest of the section will continue in effect.

Introduction

A lot of people have trouble getting pregnant, but not very many are willing to talk about it. After all, most couples are worried about conceiving unexpectedly. When you first realize that your efforts aren't working, it can be confusing and upsetting.

Infertility can be a terrible cross to bear when you desperately want a child. While the world is full of advice and support for couples who are about to have a baby, it's surprisingly silent when a couple can't conceive. You might find yourself feeling as though yours is the only family that struggles with this problem.

The reality is very different; up to a quarter of couples find that they can't conceive a child for a year or more. Between three and seven percent of the population never manage to resolve their fertility problems.

That number is decreasing, however, as the medical profession discovers more ways to help childless couples overcome their fertility difficulties. There are now many options available for people who want their own baby, from conception aids and fertility monitoring to in-vitro fertilization, or IVF.

You don't have to feel as though there are no options available for you; in fact, there's a very good chance that your doctor or a specialist could help you conceive the child you've always wanted.

Remember: there's always hope, even if you've been dealing with fertility issues for a long time. New medical advances mean that most couples that suffer from infertility will be able to overcome the obstacles and have the baby they've been dreaming about.

This book is written in simple story format in order to help you understand the most common causes of infertility and their solutions. It will help you get a detailed understanding of why a couple might experience problems with conception. You'll find out how and why things sometimes go wrong with this natural process. This book can also give you a better idea of some of the trials and emotional challenges that you might face along the way to solving your family's fertility problems.

The journey to your solution might be long. For many families, it takes several tries to overcome the challenges of infertility. This book can help serve as your guide to dealing with the trials, challenges and disappointments that sometimes stand between you and a positive pregnancy test or healthy birth.

With the right attitude, however, you and your family can make it through these obstacles. Let the story of Jennifer and Michael – a typical couple suffering from infertility – serve as your guide and help you make the right choices to help you conceive.

AN INCONCEIVABLE PROBLEM

In the beginning

Like most couples, we always assumed that we would have a baby when the time was right. There were careers to contend with and we both had to build a life together before we could even start thinking about expanding our family. That's why, once we decided to try for a baby, it took us a while to realize that something was wrong. Even though we were hoping to have a child, we never seemed to get pregnant.

All around us, our friends and family members who had recently married were having no trouble conceiving. One couple we knew from college even had twins! Our relatives started asking us when we were going to add to the family, and we didn't know what to tell them. It seemed like we must be doing something wrong, since no one else was having trouble.

After a few years, it even started to feel like other people were judging us. After all, a lot of people seem to think that women who don't have kids by the time they're 30 are selfish. We were still trying hard to have a baby, but it was too personal to talk about with everyone around us. I started to feel like I had let my husband and my family down.

Both of us began to feel very depressed and hopeless. We'd never known anyone who had this kind of problem getting pregnant. Infertility had always seemed like it was something that happened to other people. We even wondered if we simply weren't meant to have a baby.

Eventually, I got the courage to bring the subject up with my doctor. It might seem like that should have been the first thing we would do, but it took us a long time to figure things out and realize it was more than just bad luck. The idea of being unable to have the baby that we'd always wanted seemed impossible.

The doctor was puzzled, too. At first glance, we seemed like a couple that should have no trouble conceiving. We were both healthy and fit, neither of us smoked, and I had no family history of reproductive problems. After a few tests, it was clear that something was wrong, but no one was quite sure what it was. That's when our journey through infertility really began.

What My Mother Never Told Me About Conception

When we started trying to deal with our problem, I didn't know a lot about having children beyond the basics you get in health class. After all, it didn't seem to be a big deal for most people. My mom never had trouble getting pregnant, and she even had easily deliveries for all three of her kids. I simply wasn't prepared to handle the realities of infertility.

As soon as we started researching our problem, we started to learn a lot. I found out that many couples actually have trouble getting pregnant, but that there isn't much support for them. That's why no one talks about it.

I also found out that the process of having a baby isn't as foolproof as your biology textbook makes it look. There are all kinds of problems that can creep in, making it hard to get pregnant and carry the child to term.

Infertility Happens to Everyone

Getting pregnant can be challenging for many people. It's not just couples who live an unhealthy lifestyle or who have health problems that deal with infertility. In fact, my doctor told me that 10 to 15 percent of the couples who live in the United States alone deal with infertility. Worldwide, that number can go up to about 28 percent, depending on what country you live in and what kind of healthcare you have access to. That's a big problem, but no one ever seems to talk about it.

Contrary to popular belief, just about anyone can have trouble having a baby. Infertility happens to people of every race and religion. Your family could experience this problem whether you are rich or poor, straight or gay, blue-collar or well-educated professionals. The risk does go up a little if you're older or if you work in certain jobs, but that doesn't mean you've done anything wrong. Infertility isn't a punishment; it can happen to any of us, just like any other medical problem.

Having a Baby Isn't Easy

Most people think that getting pregnant is something that happens as soon as you try for a baby. In real life, however, there are actually a lot more factors. Did you know that even in completely healthy couples who aren't using any kind of birth control, there's only a 15 to 25 percent chance of pregnancy? That's because fertilization happens only about one out of every four times you try for a baby. Plus, even healthy women's bodies often reject a fertilized egg early on.

Miscarriages are also very common. About 10 to 15 percent of pregnancies end in miscarriage. A lot of the time, this happens before you even know you're pregnant. Early on, this can look like a late period. After eight weeks, the risk drops to only three percent, and it drops to one percent after sixteen weeks. That's in very healthy, young people. Those of us who are older or have any kind of problem with our reproductive systems tend to have an even higher risk.

Getting pregnant might seem easy, but it's actually pretty difficult. When I found out how low the chance of fertilization and successful pregnancy actually is, I was very surprised. My mom and my health teacher definitely never told me about that!

I realized that almost every couple has at least a few problems getting pregnant after they decide it's time for a baby. Even so, our situation was unusual. We'd waited far longer than normal to get pregnant. We were starting to get worried, but we weren't sure if we were actually infertile.

Getting the Definitions Straight

When do you call it infertility? That's one of the things that we wondered when we first realized that getting pregnant was going to be harder than it should be. After all, no one wants to spend a lot of time or money on a problem that would work itself out if they just waited a little while.

Doctors consider a couple to be infertile when they have been trying to have a baby for one year with no positive results. Most ordinary couples can become pregnant within the first six months. Even the majority of people who experience trouble are usually able to have a baby in that first year. Some of us aren't blessed with that kind of luck. It takes more than just effort to conceive the child we've always dreamed of.

It's important to remember that infertility isn't the same as sterility. Doctors use the word "infertility" to imply that the problem can be diagnosed and treated; most couples who suffer from infertility are able to get pregnant eventually. Sterility means that the problem is irreversible and permanent, something that happens to only a handful of unlucky couples.

Should the Doctor Get Involved?

Admitting your fertility problems to your doctor can be embarrassing and stressful. You might wonder if you'll be judged for not be able to have a baby. After all, about two thirds of women who don't have a baby by the time they're in their mid-30s feel discriminated against. About half of us feel ashamed and unwilling to talk about our fertility. I know that it took us a long time to bring the subject up, even though we'd been worrying for years.

If you suffer from infertility for over a year, the problem isn't very likely to fix itself. That's why you need to get help. Instead of blaming yourself or wondering if the world is against you, you'll be able to find out what's causing your infertility and get the help you need. For some couples, the fix is very simple. For us, it took a little longer, but we were eventually able to have the beautiful baby we'd always wanted.

Your doctor will be able to help you figure out if your infertility is due to health problems in the man, which account for about 40 percent of cases, or if your fertility problems are due to female reproductive issues. In a lot of cases, it's hard to have a baby because something is a little bit wrong with both partners. That adds up to a bigger challenge when those two people get together.

Take the time to think carefully about what you'll say to your doctor. You can even write it down if you want. Make sure you have plenty of time left in the visit to discuss your fertility issues. After all, no one wants to feel rushed when they're talking about something this big. You might find out that your doctor or nurse is a lot more understanding than you thought. Mine was very sympathetic and ready to help me right away.

What You Need to Know About Conception
Most of us grew up believing that getting pregnant was simple: sperm meets egg, and exactly nine months later, you have a baby. That's technically true, but it's leaving out a lot. When we first started trying to get pregnant, what I didn't know about the conception process could have filled volumes!
There are a whole lot of factors that can affect whether or not you can get pregnant, including your age, the time of month, and even what you and your partner have been eating. My doctor explained some of this to me, and I did a lot of research on my own to find out more about how I could improve my chances.

Ovulation

I found out that the factors that affect conception got started a long time before my husband and I tried to get pregnant. For instance, when you try to conceive a baby could make a really big difference in your chances of being successful. Women only ovulate once per month, usually about two weeks before their periods. The egg only survives for a day or two. If you don't get pregnant in that time, your body will get rid of it and prepare for your period.

It can be hard to predict exactly when you're going to ovulate, though. Not everyone experiences this at exactly the same time every month. Some women can feel a tiny sharp pain when their bodies release the egg, but I never noticed any difference. It's also possible to have an abnormal ovulation cycle. Sometimes the body doesn't make the right hormones for a woman to ovulate and she never has an egg ready to be fertilized.

Some women even go through early menopause and run out of eggs very early. Problems like these are why it's so important to go to your doctor and have some tests done if you think you might be infertile. If your body isn't ovulating correctly, hope and prayer might not be enough to fix the issue.

Fertilization

If the egg encounters sperm while it's waiting in the fallopian tube, it becomes fertilized. The structure of the egg changes so that no other sperm cells can enter. This is when the future baby's genes are determined, including the X and Y chromosomes. At this point, the egg is fertilized, but that doesn't mean that you're pregnant. This fertilized egg still has to make it all the way into the uterus in order to create a pregnancy. The whole time, its cells are dividing and it's working to grow very quickly, however.

Not everyone has an easy time getting that egg to be fertilized. If the man has a problem that causes him not to produce very much sperm, the right cells might never make it into the egg. That could also happen if the sperm isn't shaped right. Injuries or diseases are often responsible for this kind of fertilization problem.

You might not be able to get pregnant because of trouble with the woman's body, too. If you have endometriosis or you have ever suffered from PID (pelvic inflammatory disease), your fallopian tubes might be blocked. That could keep the sperm from getting to the egg to fertilize it.

Even an old surgery could make it impossible for the egg to get fertilized and implant properly. There are all kinds of things that could go wrong, but so many of us never hear about it. We think we've messed up, when the trouble is really just bad luck.

Implantation

If everything goes well, the egg stays in the fallopian tube for about three or four days after it gets fertilized. It divides rapidly into a whole lot of different cells. Then, it starts slowly moving down the tube and toward the uterus. When the egg gets to the uterus, it implants itself into the lining and starts to grow blood vessels. Some women get a little bit of light bleeding or spotting for a day or two when this happen. This might be the first sign that you're officially pregnant!

Around this time, the lining of your uterus wall will start to get a lot thicker. You'll also develop a plug that stays in place over your cervix until it's time for the baby to be born. Unfortunately, you can't tell that either of these things is happening. If you don't get spotting when the fertilized egg implants, you might not know that you're pregnant until you take a pregnancy test.

Pregnancy tests measure the amount of a specific hormone in your blood or urine. This hormone is called human chorionic gonadotropin, but most people just refer to it as HCG. The cells that eventually turn into the baby's placenta put this hormone out, but it takes a little while. For most of us, it can be an agonizing three to four weeks before there's enough of this hormone available to confirm that we are pregnant. By that time, the fertilized egg will have started to turn into an embryo. It will even have the very first nerve cells, but it won't look much like a baby yet.

Implantation isn't always perfect, either. A lot of normal, healthy women never experience pregnancy after fertilization occurs because the egg simply doesn't implant. It's flushed out with the next period and the cycle begins again. In those of us who have fertility problems, that can happen even more often. Every time it looks like we might get pregnant, something goes wrong and the fertilized egg isn't able to implant.

There are a lot of reasons that this might happen to you. If you engage in a whole lot of really heavy exercise while the egg is trying to implant, your body might not get the process right. If you're trying to get pregnant, it might be time to hold off on your triathlon training and postpone that half marathon. Normal exercise won't cause the same kinds of problems, so there's nothing wrong with jogging or lifting weights.

Sometimes an egg just doesn't implant. Other times, it starts to implant and something goes wrong. This is very common even in women who don't have any kind of health problem, but if you have endometriosis or your uterus is an unusual shape, you might run into even more problems with implantation. If you have any of these problems, your doctor might be able to help you with surgery.

It's still important to have your pregnancy monitored closely afterward, though. Even women who can have their bodies fixed through surgery have a higher chance of losing the pregnancy than people who never had infertility problems. It's just one of those unlucky facts!

After Pregnancy Begins

Pregnancy officially occurs at implantation, but infertility problems can continue after this point. Under normal conditions, it takes about a week for the embryo to split into two parts, creating the placenta. The next week, the baby-to-be will develop a heart. The week after that, the embryo starts to grow its own unique brain. By the time a normal pregnancy has reached week 12, the baby can move inside the uterus and is developing reflexes. This essential period is when a lot of important development happens, but it's also when many women suffer miscarriages.

About 10 to 15 percent of women who know they are pregnant still have a miscarriage, and a lot more of us experience them without ever being aware that we're carrying a baby. More than three quarters of these miscarriages happen in the first 12 weeks. They might happen because there is something wrong with the baby, or because the mother has a health issue. For instance, if you have a blood clotting disorder, you might not be able to keep a baby after 10 weeks.

Later miscarriages are also a risk. If you have scar tissue or something went wrong when your uterus and cervix developed, your body might not be able to maintain the pregnancy. You might also have problems with miscarriage if you get an infection, overuse any kind of drugs, are in an accident, or have a disease like diabetes or hypothyroidism.

These problems can be very stressful and they can happen over and over again, but it's important not to give up hope. Even those of us who have trouble conceiving or carrying a baby are often able to have the child we've always prayed for. It's just a matter of finding out what's wrong and getting the help we need.

How We Tried

Once my husband and I found out about all the different things that could be keeping us from having our baby, we decided to do something about them. We started off with the least expensive and least invasive options, hoping that something would work easily.

There are all kinds of options out there, both from doctors and from the alternative health community. Unfortunately, our journey was long and we had to try a lot of different things before we found the perfect solution to our infertility problems.

Vitamins and Timing

When we weren't able to get pregnant after the usual three or four months, we wondered if we were just doing something wrong. Maybe we didn't time things right. Maybe I didn't have enough of the right vitamins in my system to keep the baby-to-be healthy. I started taking prenatal vitamins to help make sure I had all the right nutrition to support our new child. We also started looking into ways to figure out when it would be best to try for a baby.

It turns out that if you observe the changes in your body over the course of the month, you can get a much better chance of conception. The mucus around the cervix changes to become very slippery. This makes it easier for sperm to survive inside your body. It also helps the sperm make it to the egg they need to fertilize. Your body temperature also fluctuates. You need to take your temperature every day for a little while to help you figure out when you're likely to ovulate. Normally, your temperature will be lower right before ovulation and higher right afterward.

All these calculations felt a little inconvenient, but we were willing to give them a try if it meant we had a better chance of getting pregnant. After all, my cousin hadn't been able to conceive for a few months, but once she started keeping track of things, she had a beautiful baby girl. This technique definitely works for couples who simply haven't had the luck to try for a baby on the right day.

Unfortunately, our problem turned out to be more than just bad timing or the wrong nutrition. Even after a few months of tracking my temperature and making sure we were intimate at all the right times, we still didn't have any results. It was frustrating and depressing to put all that energy into getting pregnant without anything to show for it. We didn't give up, but sometimes we were definitely tempted to.

A Question of Age

Most people know that older women have more trouble getting pregnant and having children. We started to wonder if I was too old to successfully have a baby. After all, like a lot of other people we had waited until our early 30s to try for a child. Before then, careers, money issues and a lot of other things had simply gotten in the way. We asked our doctor about it, but he said that my age was probably not the biggest problem.

About a third of couples who have their first baby after the age of 35 deal with fertility problems. That's because women start to experience changes in their reproductive organs after this age. As we get older, we have fewer eggs and our ovaries get less effective at releasing them. Many of the eggs will be unhealthy, making it harder to fertilize one successfully. That's part of why birth defects and spontaneous miscarriages happen a lot more as we get older. Plus, the more the years pass, the more likely we are to have a health problem that could get in the way of fertility.

This is why doctors have special infertility rules for couples who are a little older. If you are over the age of 35 and you have been trying to get pregnant for six months, it might be time to talk to your doctor. Waiting the extra six months for a normal diagnosis of infertility could decrease your chances even more. We were happy not to fall into this category, but we made sure to let all our friends know that this could be a problem. We didn't want anyone else to go through the nightmare of infertility alone.

All Those Tests

When we finally brought our concerns up with our doctor, there were a lot of possibilities in front of us. Both of us had to go through a bunch of different tests to rule out possible problems. A lot of them were scary and upsetting, but they were also important if we wanted to get pregnant eventually. Without all the testing, it would have been impossible to know whether we were good candidates for in vitro fertilization, the route we eventually chose to help us complete our family.

My husband went through testing to make sure that he had normal sperm production and to rule out the possibility of a disease or birth defect that was getting in the way of conception. Once the doctors ruled out the most common problems that men have, however, his job was pretty simple. Mine was a lot more complicated, and it lasted much longer.

I had to go through even more testing and questionnaires, since there are so many more things that could go wrong. For a little while, I felt like it was unfair that my husband got off relatively easily, but he was sweet and supportive the entire time. There are simply a lot more possibilities for infertility in women because we need to provide the right environment for our babies to develop properly.

My doctor checked me for polycystic ovary syndrome, or PCOS, hyperprolactinemia, tumors, hormone disorders and all kinds of other problems that can get in the way of fertilization and pregnancy. He asked me about my family history, weight fluctuations, my diet and even how many drinks I had every month. All this information got written down on my charts and brought out whenever I needed to talk to another specialist.

I didn't like going through it; it felt invasive and I worried that I might have done something to permanently keep us from having a baby. I started to hate having to go in to get yet another test done, but I tried to remember that it was all for a good cause. Eventually, all those tests could lead to having a baby of our very own.

The cost of it all made us worry, too. It turns out that most insurance plans specifically refuse to cover treatment for infertility. They think that it's "elective" instead of necessary to fix a medical problem. Most families who suffer from this issue could tell their insurers that just like a lot of the other things the companies refuse to pay for, infertility treatment is anything but optional.

Being childless when you want a baby puts a lot of strain and emotional stress on every family. It can even cause depression, anxiety, and a lot of other mental health issues. Insurers don't see it that way, however. Our doctor did what he could to code things so that they would be covered, but we ended up having to handle most of the bills on our own.

The good news is that the initial costs were relatively low, and we had time to make a budget to cover the more expensive treatments. If you think that you might have serious fertility problems, I would recommend taking the time to do your research before you start looking for treatment. No one wants to be unable to afford the cost of having a baby when the right solution is so close at hand. Later on, I'll talk a little bit more about the cost of fertility treatment and the best ways to make sure that your budget can handle it.

Searching for Answers

We spent a lot of time talking to our doctor and to other experts in order to figure out what could be wrong.

Unfortunately, it didn't turn out to be anything obvious and easy to fix. If I hadn't been ovulating correctly, for instance, I could have taken some medications that would make sure that I had an egg available when we were trying for a baby.

If my body wasn't producing the right kind of mucus for fertilization, the doctor could have given me a drug designed to make this easier. Some couples who have this problem or other ovulation issues actually have healthy sperm placed right in the uterus around the time of ovulation. That keeps any physical issues the couple might have from getting in the way of healthy conception.

This only works for women who can carry a baby normally once the egg has been fertilized, however. If you have scars in your uterus or other problems, this kind of treatment might not be ideal for you.

If we had experienced any of these relatively straightforward problems, we might have been candidates for these types of infertility treatments. Unfortunately, it turned out that our issues were a little bit more complicated. In fact, the doctor couldn't figure out what was wrong right away. We were diagnosed as suffering from infertility with unknown causes.

That's not all that uncommon. About 20 percent of the infertile couples in the US alone have unexplained infertility. It's not something you hear much about, but it is a real thing. That doesn't mean that there aren't reasons for us to have trouble conceiving. It just means that medical science isn't yet advanced enough for doctors to know why the problem occurs.

Unexplained infertility has all kinds of possible causes, but no one has determined which ones are most likely to be the culprits. Not knowing can make things seem pretty intimidating, but it won't keep you from having a baby forever.

Just because your infertility doesn't have a clear explanation doesn't mean that you can't get help, however. A lot of couples who have trouble getting pregnant but don't know why are still able to eventually have a baby. They simply have to use more advanced techniques to help them overcome their unknown problems. That's the category that we fell into. Eventually we were able to have our child, but there were many hurdles to get past before our happy ending. With the help of supportive medical professionals and friends, we were able to make it through everything!

Choosing IVF

Once we knew that the more basic treatments for infertility weren't going to work for us, it was time to start doing some research. We needed help from specialists who had a lot of experience with infertile couples. They were able to help us pick out a more advanced option that could help us conceive.

There are several different kinds of advanced infertility treatments available. The most common, and the one that ended up working for us, is called in vitro fertilization, or IVF. It involves collecting eggs and sperm from the couple, then fertilizing the egg outside the body. Your doctor might also call it ART, for assisted reproductive technology. That's the broader category of advanced treatment that IVF belongs to, and it contains a few other similar treatments.

Because I wasn't able to successfully create and sustain a pregnancy, we needed the help of doctors to make sure the process worked correctly. By fertilizing the eggs outside of my body and implanting them directly into my womb, we were able to successfully have a happy and healthy baby without the repeated failures and disappointments that had always been part of our efforts.

Getting IVF wasn't smooth sailing the whole way through, however. It's an involved process and there aren't any guarantees. We worried that we might be wasting money on something that might not work. The process itself can be pretty uncomfortable, too. The doctor and specialists were friendly and happy to give us a lot of information about what to expect, though. Just knowing what might and might not happen helped us feel a lot better about our prospects of having a baby together.

IVF Basics

Most people who use IVF have one of two problems. Either the mother-to-be has problems with her fallopian tubes or the potential father has trouble with sperm quality. We didn't have either of those issues, but we still qualified. That's because couples with unexplained infertility who haven't conceived after a few years may be encouraged to try IVF. In the UK, the official rules of the medical system even recommend it for people in our situation. In the US and other countries, it tends to depend on your doctor. If you're not sure whether IVF might be an option for you, don't be afraid to ask!

The term "in vitro" means outside the body. It usually refers to processes that take place in a medical or scientific lab, like tests that kill cancer cells in a test tube. That's why the first babies conceived with the help of IVF were often called "test tube babies." That might make you think about babies who were born entirely artificially, but it really only refers to a fertilization process that happens outside the womb.

By fertilizing the egg in the lab, doctors can control its environment and prevent outside factors from getting in the way. They don't have to deal with anatomical problems, hormonal issues, or regular old bad luck. They do need to get the reproductive cells outside the parents' bodies, though. For men, this is usually pretty simple, but women have a more difficult time.

There are four major types of IVF. They're distinguished by how the doctors collect egg cells from the mother. The first one is called natural IVF. The first test tube babies were born using this technique. It involves collecting eggs as part of the woman's natural menstrual cycle. That makes it a lot less invasive and decreases the risk of side effects.

Unfortunately, natural IVF is a lot less effective. Older mothers between the ages of 40 and 42 have only a 1.3 percent success rate using this method. It is a good idea for people who need to avoid the side effects of taking drugs, however.

If you want to use a relatively natural method but can't deal with the low success rate, you can also choose modified natural IVF or mild IVF. These both involve using medications, but they're designed to reduce the risk of problems. Modified natural IVF calls for the medication to be used just a couple of days per month.

It reduces the risk of an egg appearing too quickly. It also provides more eggs to work with. It's the most popular kind of natural technique and it works really well for women who don't have very many eggs left in their ovaries.

People who can tolerate a little more medication can try mild IVF. This involves using a small dose of ovarian stimulating drugs during a short. It still relies on the natural cycle for collection and it doesn't have very many side effects. If you use mild IVF, you'll only get two to seven eggs. The goal is to produce as many healthy embryos as possible from as few eggs as possible.

A little more than 40 percent of pregnancies that use this technique result in live births. That's slightly less effective than normal, medication-based methods. This method is also a little cheaper and reduces your risk of having twins, triplets or more, but it can be hard to find a doctor to help you with it.

Conventional IVF is the most widespread method and it's the one we ended up using. It has the highest success rate, which means that about 45 percent of pregnancies from conventional IVF end in live birth. It does use a higher dose of medicine to make sure that your ovaries produce plenty of eggs. There are also some other medications involved to keep you from ovulating at the wrong time. If you use what is called "short protocol" conventional IVF, you might skip those medications, but it raises the risk of early or late ovulation.

The doctors monitor your hormone levels the whole time. They also take sonograms to check on your progress. You have to get injections for about 10 days, which can be difficult for some people. This method is common and has been tested for a very long time, though. It's also the most effective kind of IVF. If you use conventional methods, you should know that you have a higher risk of twins, triplets or even more! For some of us, that's an added bonus, but for families who are only ready for one baby it can be a stressful surprise.

Collecting the Eggs

Whether you use ovulation stimulating drugs or you do it naturally, the doctor will still need to collect them. They normally give you a trigger shot of hCG that makes you ovulate within three days. A little before the eggs would normally release, the doctors collect them with a needle. It takes about 20 to 40 minutes and you need anesthetic before the procedure, but it's pretty safe.

The needle does have to go through your vaginal wall to reach the ovaries. That can be pretty scary. It can also hurt for a little while after the anesthetic wears off. When the process is done, the doctors will have as many as 20 egg cells to work with. That raises your chance of eventually having a viable pregnancy and a healthy child.

Everything went well for me and I was just a little sore afterwards, but some people do have trouble. If you have PCOS and not a lot of body fat, you might develop a hemorrhage. Some unlucky women also get an infection after the procedure, but this isn't very common. Doctors have been using this technique since the mid-1980s and they've had a lot of time to practice!

In the Lab

After doctors collect enough eggs, they'll also ask the man for a sample of his sperm. He usually has things a lot easier! The lab technicians strip any surrounding cells off of the eggs and prepare them for fertilization. Sometimes they analyze the eggs to see which ones are most likely to produce healthy babies. This can cost more and might make the process more complicated, though.

The lab will also remove any extra cells and fluid from the

father's contribution. They put the two kinds of cells together in a culture medium and incubated it for anywhere from one to 24 hours, depending on the lab. The warm temperatures and culture medium imitate the conditions inside the human body, making it a lot more likely for fertilization to occur. If the sperm count is low or the sperm are damaged, the technicians might inject one cell into an egg to make sure everything goes the way it's supposed to.

When the egg cell starts dividing, the specialists know that fertilization is complete. They move it to a special growth medium and leave it there for about two days. Over the course of that time, it will double several times. The result is just six to eight cells, but it has the potential to become a whole lot more. Some doctors choose to implant the fertilized egg at this state. Others allow the egg to divide even more, until it reaches what is known as the blastocyst stage. At this point, the egg has an outer and an inner layer of cells, or about 100 cells total. It isn't even an embryo yet, but it has a better chance of surviving than the three day old eggs used in some programs.

Almost every IVF program produces more than one embryo. Even under controlled conditions in the lab, it's too easy for a single fertilized egg to die or become damaged. A specialist will examine all the possible candidates and pick the one or ones that are most likely to survive inside the womb. Even the healthiest people often have fertilized eggs that will never turn into a baby, so it's important to rule those out early on.

Implanting Our Pregnancy

We spent a lot of time anxiously waiting around while our cells fertilized each other and developed into little clusters of potential life. Then we had to wait for the specialists to decide whether any of these cells were good enough to produce a healthy pregnancy. Eventually, the big day came. Doctors did an embryo transfer, moving the fertilized cells into my body, where they would hopefully turn into lively, growing babies.

I had to take hormones to make sure that my womb would be ready to receive those cells. Most doctors use estrogen for the first two weeks, then a combination of that hormone with progesterone to prepare the uterine lining. There's a short implantation window after the lining becomes ready. That's when the doctors implanted our embryos.

The whole process was a lot easier than trying to donate the eggs. I didn't even need anesthesia. The embryos were put into a flexible catheter and simply injected. The doctors used an ultrasound to make sure that they put the cells in the right place.

If you go through the IVF procedure, doctors will usually inject more than one set of cells. That's because only a small percentage of the fertilized eggs will actually implant. At one time, they used as many eggs as possible to increase the chance of a viable pregnancy. This has bad side effects, though. You could end up pregnant with too many babies; people who have had IVF can end up having as many as seven or eight in some cases. That's hard on your body and it could risk the health of your children.

Most countries and medical associations limit the number of embryos that doctors can use in one try. For instance, in Australia, Canada, New Zealand and the UK, doctors can implant only two at a time. If the woman is over 40 and lives in the UK, she might have up to three transferred. US patients don't have the same kind of regulations, so the number you'll receive is up to your program. Talk with your doctor about the risk of multiple births before your implantation takes place. That way, you'll know if you might have twins. If you don't use all the embryos the first time, you can have them frozen for possible future attempts.

Time to Wait and Hope

After I received the embryos, everything was over for a little while. We just had to wait to find out whether or not I was going to get pregnant. Even the best cases of IVF only have about a 50 percent rate of pregnancy. The older you get, the harder it is to get pregnant, too. At 35, the rate goes down to about 40 percent. By the time you're over 40, the rate of successful pregnancy is as low as 20 percent. Miscarriage rates are higher, too. Only about 12 percent of women over 40 who get IVF have a successful birth.

We weren't too old, but all those figures made us feel very nervous. Would our embryo implant? Would we be able to get through the pregnancy without running into more problems? It was a very scary time, but eventually we got the good news. Our pregnancy test was positive!

Other Forms of ART

Not everyone will use IVF, but most people will need something similar. There are several other forms of ART that might work, depending on your specific situation. Some of them are very similar to IVF, but they use slightly different techniques that can make them more effective or less invasive for certain people.

One option is ZIFT, or zygote intrafallopian transfer. This works a lot like IVF, but the implantation process is different. Just like with IVF, the doctors combine sperm and egg cells outside the uterus. After the cells are fertilized, however, they are transferred to the fallopian tubes, just like a natural pregnancy.
The big benefit of using ZIFT is that it has a slightly higher success rate. It requires at least one fallopian tube to be normal, though, so ZIFT isn't an option if you have extensive scarring or other issues. It's best for people who have already tried other techniques with no beneficial results. As IVF has improved, the number of ZIFT procedures has gone down, but some people still use this technique to get the child they have always wanted.

GIFT is a similar procedure. The letters stand for gamete intrafallopian transfer In fact, it's the one that doctors developed ZIFT from. It involves transferring the sperm and the eggs directly into the fallopian tube. The fertilization and implantation happen naturally from there. GIFT is an older technique that takes four to six weeks to complete. It produces results in about a third of cases and is best for couples who have trouble with sperm cells or who just don't know why they're infertile.

Most people use IVF instead of GIFT because it is easier and less invasive. Some couples don't like the idea of fertilization and embryo growth happening in the lab, however. GIFT is the most natural form of ART and is more compatible with some people's religious beliefs.

When there is a big problem with the man's ability to produce viable cells, doctors sometimes use ICSI, or intracytoplasmic sperm injection. This is also sometimes used in cases where the couple is older and has already tried IVF with no success. The sperm is injected directly into the egg, then the IVF procedure continues normally.

When Your Body Isn't Enough

If you or your partner has a reproductive problem that would normally prevent you from getting pregnant at all, you don't have to give up hope. It's very possible to get the assistance of someone else, whether it's a sperm or egg donor or a surrogate, to help you conceive a child. For instance, if you know that you can't easily produce fertile eggs, the contents of a fertile egg from a donor can be placed into one of your infertile eggs. Then the doctor uses ICSI to fertilize it. This way, you can carry a child made up of some of your shared genetic material, but with the help of a donor.

If the father has trouble producing viable sperm cells, it might be appropriate to use a donor for this, too. You can choose from anonymous donors, donors with known histories, or even a friend of the family. While the baby's genetics might be a little different from what you might hope, it's a good way to overcome infertility and build the family you've always wanted.

You might also experience a situation where your reproductive cells are perfectly viable, but you can't or shouldn't carry a baby to term. Some women have to have their uteruses removed due to cancer or other problems, but still have working ovaries. Others suffer from conditions that could make a pregnancy very dangerous. You might even be able to get pregnant, but multiple miscarriages make it very hard to have a life birth.

That's when a surrogate can help. Gestational surrogacy involves all the same IVF techniques we used to conceive our child, but the embryo is implanted into the womb of a surrogate mother. She carries the child to birth, but you are the real parents. Surrogacy can be expensive, but it's a legitimate way to have a genetically related child when you can't otherwise carry a baby.

Try, Try Again

We were very lucky. Our first attempt at IVF helped us conceive and carry a healthy baby to term. That's beating the odds, since up to two thirds of parents who use IVF don't succeed on the first try. That's why it's so important to have extra embryos frozen if you use a method that produces multiple fertilized eggs. That way, you can try once more without the need to go through the ovulation and collection process all over again.

It's normal to have trouble conceiving with IVF. After all, this is a difficult process at best, and sometimes nature takes its course. You just have to be willing to try again or use a different technique in order to get things right. It can be heartbreaking to hear that you weren't able to conceive the first time, but patience could help you have the baby of your dreams.

If you're willing to talk about the situation with your doctor and even get a second opinion, you'll have an easier time staying informed about your options. Treating infertility can be a scary process, it's true, but your family will be happier and bigger if you're willing to stick with it.

When Getting Pregnant Seems Worse Than Infertility

When you're going through the IVF process, sometimes it can seem like it's actually worse than experiencing infertility. I know that I felt as though I had given up my right to any kind of privacy. Doctors and other specialists were asking me all kinds of questions about my sex life, my body and other very private subjects. I had to submit to regular testing, and for a while it even felt like I was spending more time at the clinic than at home!

The reason I'm talking about this is because almost everyone who has reproductive therapy feels like things are impossible at some point. Even though IVF and other treatments are pretty effective, they aren't fast or easy. Friends and family might wonder why you're not excited to have found a solution. Even your best supporters can have trouble understanding.

The key is to make sure that you keep your goal in sight and remember to take care of yourself. It's normal to feel frustrated, anxious and even depressed when you're undergoing this kind of treatment. I eventually decided to see a counselor to help me deal with all the added stress. She was able to help me keep the reasons for these treatments in focus and avoid letting all the difficulties get in the way.

I also made sure to create time for me and my husband together as a couple. All the impersonal questions and invasive procedures of IVF can make it hard to feel good about being intimate together. Even if you're not interested in having sex or the doctor tells you to avoid it, you can still spend quality time together and make sure you get plenty of hugs, kisses and cuddling. It'll help reinforce your bonds as a family and it'll reduce stress for both of you.

Another important thing in the face of IVF treatment is making time for yourself. Let yourself relax and forget about all the stressful things in your life for a little while every week. Take care of your body so that you'll feel good about yourself. I know that the amount of time I spent in a little paper robe was definitely a blow to my self esteem. If you're willing to take care of yourself, however, all the problems of dealing with infertility will fade into the background for a little while.

We thought our journey through infertility would be easier once we found the right solution, but it actually became even harder to deal with for a little while. We finally began to hope that we might really have a baby, but the idea that it might not work was really stressful. Learning to relieve our stress and keep focused on the reason we were doing everything was essential to getting through it all.

Section title 5.1

To our dismay, getting pregnant wasn't the end of our infertility journey. Couples who have experienced problems with conception often experience higher-risk pregnancies. We tend to be older or have complicated health situations that mean more monitoring. I spent a lot of time in the doctor's office while I was carrying our son!

This period was almost as confusing and worrying as trying to get pregnant had been. I didn't have much guidance from women in my family, since most of them had experienced normal pregnancies. No one really tells you what you should expect when you're carrying a child conceived through reproductive therapy. I'll talk a little bit about my experience here so that you'll have an easier time than I did. There are lots of tests and some extra drugs that you might need, and it's worth it to know what you might encounter.

Progesterone Support

After the implantation process, your doctor might keep you on progesterone support. This hormone is important in any pregnancy, but it can be vital in women who have a history of hormonal disruption or who have conceived through IVF. The Fertility Care Centers of America note that a lot of women who have spontaneous miscarriages in the first trimester experience lower progesterone levels. Supplementing your hormones helps decrease the risk of this tragedy throughout your pregnancy.

Blood Testing

I also had to get my hormone levels checked on a regular basis. That meant a lot of trips to the doctor to get blood tests. They made sure that my hCG, or pregnancy hormone, levels were rising but not too high. If your levels stay low, it might mean that the baby isn't healthy. If they get too high, you might be carrying twins or more. Since multiple pregnancies are riskier, doctors try to avoid them after infertility treatments.

The tests also kept track of my estrogen levels. That's important because some women can develop a problem after IVF treatment. It's called ovarian hyperstimulation syndrome, or OHSS. This only happens to about one in 10 patients, but it can be dangerous.

When OHSS happens, the ovaries become enlarged and can leak into the chest and belly. You might gain weight, feel bloated, feel nauseated or have stomach problems. In serious cases, you could feel dizzy or have a rapid heartbeat. OHSS usually goes away on its own, but some patients might have to go to the hospital to have fluid removed. The good news is that there are ways to stop this from happening while you're receiving the IVF treatment, and monitoring your estrogen levels during the first part of pregnancy will make sure your health stays stable.

Ultrasounds

Eventually, your fertility doctor will probably transfer you to your regular gynecologist or obstetrician. Before this happens, however, he or she is going to have to make sure that the pregnancy is healthy and stable. You'll need one or two ultrasounds during the early part of your pregnancy to check for multiple implantations and make sure that everything is progressing the way that it should. You might get to see your baby's heartbeat on the ultrasound if the scans occur during the right week.

Talking to Your Normal Obstetrician

Most IVF pregnancies progress normally after the initial stages are over. If your pregnancy doesn't seem to be especially high-risk, you'll be able to deal directly with a normal OB after about the second month of pregnancy. This might help relieve some of your financial pressures, since many insurers cover pregnancy but don't handle fertility treatments. It can also help you feel more comfortable since you're seeing a "normal" medical professional instead of a fertility specialist.

I actually had a little bit of trouble adjusting when I started seeing my old OB/GYN again after so many visits to the fertility specialist. After all, the IVF process was very intensive. I had to be monitored almost constantly to make sure everything was going smoothly. Seeing the obstetrician just once a month made me worry that something bad was going to happen to me or the baby.

When I brought up my fears, however, the doctor was really understanding. She suggested an additional ultrasound to make certain that everything was still okay. She knew that I'd gone through a lot to get this pregnancy and that I was willing to do a lot more to keep it.

The ultrasound showed no abnormalities, and it calmed my nerves and made me feel much safer. Once you start to receive treatment from your obstetrician, your pregnancy should progress normally, ending in delivery less than a year later. You might have a natural delivery or a C-section, just like anyone else, and you'll soon be holding your own little bundle of joy.

High Risk Pregnancies

If your fertility doctor decides that your pregnancy falls into the "high-risk" category, that doesn't mean you won't have your baby. It does mean that you won't be transferred to your normal obstetrician, however. You'll need to see a specialist called a high-risk obstetrician. This doctor knows how to deal with complicated pregnancies and is capable of helping you through difficult times to a healthy delivery.

There are a few reasons that you might be classified as higher-risk. For instance, if you already have another health problem like diabetes or high blood pressure, it could raise the chance of problems with the baby. Cancer survivors, people who have epilepsy, and survivors of kidney disease can also fall into this category. You'll need extra help to manage the condition safely while still having a healthy and stable pregnancy.

Anyone who smokes, drinks regularly or uses illegal drugs is also considered high risk, but not very many people who pursue IVF use these substances. Most of us spend a lot of time trying to be as healthy as possible in the hope of getting pregnant the natural way.

New moms who are older than 35 might be considered to have higher risk levels than people who are a little younger. Multiple pregnancies and anyone who has already had three or more miscarriages also qualify. All these situations require delicate handling to make sure that the baby or babies reach birth safely.

Not all high-risk pregnancies are associated with new parents, either. If an ultrasound shows that your baby might have a genetic problem or a birth defect, you'll need to talk to a specialist. The same thing applies if you've been pregnant before and had a problem then, even if you never delivered. Make sure you talk to your doctor about any health problems you've had and your past history. Don't be tempted to hide cases of early labor or miscarriage in the hope that you won't be classified as high-risk; seeing the specialist is a good thing, not a punishment. It'll help you make sure that you do everything right while you're carrying your baby.

If you're seeing a high-risk obstetrician, you'll go to the doctor more often. Instead of visiting once a month, you might return to the office every two or three weeks. You might also need to have more ultrasound tests to check on the health of your baby. The doctor will check your blood pressure more and do more blood and urine tests to make sure that everything is going well.

If you're older or have ever had a problem with a pregnancy, you might also have genetic tests performed to make sure that your child will be healthy. Not all high-risk pregnancies will require extremely intensive care, though. Sometimes the doctor's job will just involve making sure that you can safely take your medicine without hurting your baby. It all depends on your particular situation. Make sure to ask any extra questions you have. Being informed is essential!

Affording IVF and ART

No one plans to be infertile. That's why the cost of infertility treatments can come as such a surprise. In the United States, most insurance companies exclude coverage for medical treatments related to infertility. That puts the financial burden for this legitimate health problem on couples that are already experiencing a lot of stress and sadness. Many would-be parents feel like financial pressures will keep them from having a baby entirely. We certainly felt a lot of strain when we built our budget for infertility treatment.

You don't have to let the high costs of IVF and other reproductive therapies keep you from having a child, however. There are ways to improve your situation, make the treatments a little more economical, and save up enough to let you afford a pregnancy. It does take some advance planning, so it's a good idea to start thinking about the possibilities at the first sign of trouble. It could save some valuable time and increase your chances of a healthy pregnancy.

Can I Get Coverage?

Not all insurers deny coverage for couples that have reproductive problems. According to the National Infertility Association, some states actually mandate comprehensive insurance coverage that includes infertility treatment. They include California, Illinois, Connecticut, Massachusetts, Texas and about nine others. If you are lucky enough to live in one of these states, you may already have coverage. Ask your insurer to find out more.

Couples who live outside the United States might also be able to receive discounted or free infertility treatments as long as they meet the right criteria. In the UK, reproductive therapy clinics are monitored by the HFEA, which also sets guidelines for treatment. You can receive IVF if you have been trying for a baby for at least two years without success. Similar conditions apply in much of Europe, Australia and New Zealand, and other countries with a national health care system. Japan actively encourages women to receive infertility treatments.

Even in areas where insurers frequently deny claims relating to infertility, things may change. The United States' Affordable Care Act has changed the minimum requirements for insurance coverage. It allows doctors to offer treatments such as IVF earlier, so that couples don't have to waste time and money trying less effective treatments that cost less. The act does not mandate coverage for infertility, but it encourages it indirectly.

Many insurers will add coverage for reproductive therapies based on this act, but that doesn't mean that all plans will be the same. Grandfathered plans, large group plans and plans for the self-insured don't have to conform to these rules. When in doubt, ask your insurer. More and more medical professionals are coming to realize that infertility treatment is a legitimate therapy for real medical problems, not an optional elective choice. You could be surprised by your ability to get coverage.

The Cost of Reproductive Therapy

If you receive any kind of coverage or assistance for your infertility treatments, the amount you pay will depend on your insurer or local healthcare system. If you're footing the bill yourself, however, you should know what to expect before you jump in. Like many other medical treatments, the cost of reproductive care can be extremely high. By keeping track of normal prices, you can determine whether your hospital or clinic's charges are fair and shop around for the best providers.

IVF costs are figured based on a single care cycle. One cycle includes monthly monitoring, ovarian stimulation, harvesting and fertilizing eggs, and implanting the resulting embryos. According to the American Society for Reproductive Medicine, you can expect the cost of one cycle to average about $12,000. Depending on where you live and what your circumstances might be, this could range anywhere from $8,000 to $15,000, though. We were lucky enough to find a good doctor who charged somewhat less than average, so we didn't have to completely destroy our savings just to have a family.

You don't have to jump right into another full cycle if the first set of implantations doesn't work, however. It only costs $2,000 to $4,000 to freeze embryos for a second set of implantations, which can give you another chance without the need for a new IVF cycle. If you're insured, this is the area your provider is least likely to cover.

Smart Planning for Fertility Treatments

These average costs aren't necessarily all the average couple will be expected to pay. Tests, drugs and other necessities can add up unexpectedly, and your clinic or doctor might not tell you up front. Be willing to ask about the costs and billing for any treatments you receive.

Remember that your doctor isn't trying to scam you; he or she is focused on your reproductive health and your ability to build a family. Many doctors aren't even aware of what their services and facilities could cost their patients. By asking in advance, you can minimize unnecessary or redundant treatments and make sure that you're using only what you need, when you need it.

Decide whether or not you're willing to make big changes to your life in order to conceive. Some will choose to take out a loan, allowing them to save precious time and have a baby sooner. You might decide to move to a state where insurers are required to cover your treatments or look for a job where infertility benefits are part of the package. It might even be appropriate to use retirement money or other rainy day savings, as long as you know you can replace them once your child is born.

We had to ask ourselves questions about all of these things when the medical bills started to pile up. Once our friends and family found out about our woes, they were willing to help us; we even started a contribution fund to make sure that we could afford our first IVF cycle.

Consider talking to your family members or getting donations from people you know. There are online contribution services designed especially to help with situations just like this. It could mean the difference between having your child and continuing to wait.

Building a Budget

If you think infertility treatment might be necessary, it's time to start taking a look at your budget. A lot of financial planners recommend using the 60 percent rule to set aside money for situations like this. The basic idea is to use 60 percent of your income for essentials like food, clothing, shelter and taxes. The remaining 40 percent can go to savings, debt repayment and entertainment. If you can get your essential expenses down to 60 percent of your income, the amount you have available to help you build a family increases dramatically.

Remember to talk to your partner about this, however. He or she might be taken by surprise if you make financial decisions without a long and detailed conversation. It could even put stress on your relationship. Trying to have a baby is often difficult enough; so don't add more problems by failing to think through your financial decisions.

When we put together our budget, we found a lot of things that we could cut back on or do without in the short term. After all, once we made it through the infertility treatment process, we wouldn't have to scrimp and save for our healthcare anymore. For a little while, we made our coffee at home, ate out once a month, and made do with last years' clothes and older cars and phones. It wasn't a lot of fun, but it was easy compared to all the stress of waiting and hoping with no results.

What we didn't let our tighter budget do was eating into the essentials. It's one thing to give up some extras in order to afford reproductive treatment, but it's another to tighten your food budget or end up worrying about the electric bill. Affording IVF can seem difficult, but putting too much pressure on your bank account can also increase your stress as a couple. That makes conceiving even more difficult. Many women will fail to ovulate when they're under a lot of stress.

Flexibility

Advance planning and research can only help so much. After all, the world of infertility is unpredictable and complex. You could get pregnant earlier than you expect, or you might end up having to try multiple times. You need to build some flexibility into your plans and expectations in order to make sure your attempts will be a success.

We were aware that many couples need more than one cycle of IVF in order to get pregnant. One thing we did was to look into the possibility of financing programs that offered a refund if the treatment wasn't successful. We also talked to our financial advisor to find out what our borrowing options might be and whether our strategies were a good idea.

This extra flexibility didn't end up being necessary in our case, but it made the process of budgeting a lot less stressful. We knew that we weren't putting all our eggs in one basket and that if something went wrong, we still had options.

ONE HAPPY FAMILY

After what felt like a long and difficult journey, our dreams finally came true. We have a beautiful, healthy son through the miracle of IVF, and our family finally feels complete. When I look back on all the costs, the stress and the medical treatments, all I can think is that everything we went through was worthwhile. It was really difficult during some parts of our infertility journey, but simply having our baby made it all fade into the background.

Not everyone will have the same path through the difficulties of infertility. Some couples will be able to conceive simply by monitoring their bodies and continuing to try for a baby. Others will get pregnant after a little bit of hormonal assistance from their doctors.

A lot of couples are just like us, however. They find out that IVF is the key to their infertility woes. It might take two or more cycles, but this safe, reliable technique can be a great help. For my husband and I and couples just like us, in vitro fertilization has been the beginning of a loving, close-knit family.

Today, we're raising our son and enjoying watching all his firsts. Soon it'll be time to think about sending him to his first day of school. These are all things we'd never have experienced if we had been too afraid to mention our fertility problems to the doctor. The process was long and difficult, but it was worth it in the end to see my happy family together!

CONCLUSION

Does your situation resemble Jennifer's? Have you been waiting and hoping to have a baby without any luck? The answer could be very simple. You and thousands of other childless couples can overcome your infertility problems with the right medical help. The process takes some time and it isn't perfect, but it does have a fairly high success rate and a long history of helping people become parents.

If you've been wishing and praying to conceive for 12 months or more, it might be time to take action. You have the power to get your fertility back under control and build your own healthy family. With so many advances in medical science available, most infertile couples will find an option to help them have the child they've always wanted.

Take the time to learn about all the different possibilities. Talk to your doctor about whether IVF and other reproductive therapies might be right for you. They could help you have a child of your own after a surprisingly short wait.

No one should have to suffer from the doubt, confusion and sadness that come with infertility. We have the ability to overcome this issue, no matter what might be the cause. Every couple that wants children deserves the right to have them and see them grow up happy. Talk to your doctor today, so you can take the right steps to make your family truly complete.

Getting Pregnant Through IVF: Questions and Answers

If you've been suffering through infertility, you might feel confused by all the technical terminology your doctors throw around. This guide is designed to answer some of the most common questions you might have about in vitro fertilization and the process of overcoming your fertility issues. It'll help you feel more confident about the choices you have in front of you and allow you to make the right decision about your future family.

1. What is in vitro fertilization (IVF)?

In vitro fertilization is a fancy way of saying "fertilization in the lab." It's a series of techniques that doctors use to create a viable fertilized egg when there are problems with normal "in vivo" or "in the body" processes. They unite eggs from the mother and sperm from the father in a controlled environment and allow the eggs to grow. Then the healthiest embryos are transferred back to the mother, where they will hopefully implant and grow.

2. How many kinds of IVF are there?

Right now, there are four major types of IVF. Conventional in vitro fertilization, natural IVF, modified natural and mild

IVF. The biggest difference between them is the amount of medication used and the number of eggs that are collected. Conventional IVF uses a lot of drugs to stimulate ovulation and control your cycle. It also involves collecting a lot of eggs at once. Natural IVF doesn't use any drugs and captures only a few eggs. Mild IVF is somewhere in between the other two, while modified natural methods rely on as few drugs as possible but aren't completely drug-free. Natural and mild IVF are good for women who have problems with the medications used in normal IVF, or for people who have ethical concerns.

3. Can everyone have IVF?

In vitro fertilization helps many couples achieve the pregnancy that they've always dreamed of, but it's not right for everyone. Couples who have a poor chance of conception or who suffer from medical problems that might make IVF unsafe could be denied this treatment. If you are older than your mid-30s or have certain reproductive defects, IVF might not be right for you. On the other hand, if you suffer from PCOS, have minor uterine issues, or have a partner with low sperm count, this procedure could help you a lot.

4. Just what is PCOS?

PCOS, or polycystic ovarian syndrome, is one of the most common causes of infertility in women. It involves many tiny cysts that form in the ovaries, along with high levels of testosterone and other androgens. If you have this problem, you might develop unwanted body hair and have irregular periods. You might also have trouble ovulating normally or suffer from frequent miscarriages. IVF is a good way to bypass some of the most common fertility problems associated with

PCOS.

5. Does IVF always work?

While every infertile couple would like a "magic bullet" that definitely leads to the birth of a child, actual results aren't that good. The average success rate for couples under 35 is about 40 percent. That means one in ten tries will result in a live birth. That number goes down the older you are. Most people need more than one attempt to succeed in a live pregnancy, so don't lose hope if your first try doesn't work out. IVF is still one of the most effective options for treating infertility!

HERE ARE SOME USEFUL AND AUTHORITATIVE LINKS:

---

http://www.theafa.org/article/destination-ivf/

http://www.theafa.org/article/what-does-normal-mean-to-children-of-ivf/

http://www.theafa.org/article/what-is-in-vitro-fertilization-ivf/

http://www.theafa.org/article/how-to-understand-and-evaluate-ivf-statistics-and-success-rates/

http://www.theafa.org/blog/infertility-questions-from-readers/

http://www.theafa.org/article/how-to-give-and-receive-an-injection-a-guide-for-infertility-patients-and-their-partners/

http://www.theafa.org/article/destination-ivf/

http://www.theafa.org/article/destination-ivf/

http://www.mayoclinic.org/diseases-conditions/female-infertility/basics/treatment/con-20033618

http://www.mayoclinic.org/tests-procedures/in-vitro-fertilization/basics/definition/prc-20018905

http://www.mayo.edu/research/clinical-trials/cts-00103979

http://www.mayoclinic.org/diseases-conditions/infertility/basics/treatment/con-20034770

http://www.resolve.org/family-building-options/donor-options/after-ivf-the-embryo-decision.html

http://www.resolve.org/family-building-options/embryo-transfer-in-ivf.html

http://www.resolve.org/national-infertility-awareness-week/myths-about-iui-art-ivf.html

www.ingramcontent.com/pod-product-compliance
Lightning Source LLC
Chambersburg PA
CBHW071330310526
45789CB00017B/2167